NAVINGATING NOOM

A COMPREHENSIVE GUIDE TO BEHAVIOR CHANGES AND SUSTAINABLE WEIGHT LOSS

AHMED .R

Contents

CHAPTER ONE

INTRODUCTION

Noom is a full-service wellness program designed to assist people in reaching their fitness and health objectives by combining technology, psychology, and individualized coaching. With a focus on behavioral and psychological components of healthy living and weight loss, Noom takes a comprehensive approach to weight management, unlike standard diet plans that just emphasize calorie tracking or restrictive eating.

Important Elements of Noom:

Behavioral Change: The fundamental tenet of Noom is that long-term, sustainable weight loss and behavior modification may be attained by taking tiny, regular steps. The program's main goals are to assist participants in creating durable lifestyle changes, better habits, and mental adjustments.

Personalized Coaching: Noom gives customers access to a personal coach who will accompany them on their path and provide accountability, direction, and support. Coaches assist clients in overcoming obstacles, setting realistic objectives, and maintaining motivation. They are trained in behavior modification approaches.

Education and Awareness: To assist users in developing a deeper comprehension of psychology, fitness, and nutrition, Noom provides articles, interactive content, and educational resources. Users can make better decisions and build healthier habits by becoming more aware of the world and possessing more knowledge.

Food Tracking: Noom has a function called "Food Tracking" that uses color coding (green, yellow, and red) to classify foods according to their nutritional content and calorie density. This enables consumers to choose healthier foods without feeling constrained or undernourished.

Physical Activity: By establishing individualized activity objectives and offering advice on how to stay active, Noom helps users integrate physical activity into their everyday routines. It is believed that physical activity is crucial to general health and wellbeing.

Community Support: Noom provides a friendly environment for users to interact with one another, exchange stories, and acknowledge accomplishments. Support from the community can offer accountability, inspiration, and encouragement, making the path to improved health and fitness more pleasurable and long-lasting.

The Operation of Noom:

Assessment: First, users fill out a thorough questionnaire about their goals, lifestyle habits, preferences, and medical history. This data is utilized to generate a customized plan and personalize the program.

Goal Setting: Using the findings of the assessment, users collaborate with their personal coach to establish measurable objectives pertaining to behavior modification, physical activity, diet, and weight loss. The process of breaking down goals into small, doable steps boosts confidence and success.

Daily Assignments and Challenges: To assist users in reaching their objectives and encouraging behavior modification, Noom provides them daily assignments, challenges, and articles. These exercises concentrate on subjects like portion control, stress reduction, mindful eating, and creating healthy habits.

Tracking Progress: Using the Noom app, users may keep tabs on their weight, physical activity, food intake, and goal progress. To assist users in tracking their progress and staying on course, the app offers insights, visualizations, and comments.

Coaching and help: Individual users receive continuous help and direction from their personal coach, who follows up on a regular basis to offer encouragement, comments, and answers to queries. Coaches assist clients in navigating difficulties, overcoming roadblocks, and acknowledging accomplishments along the way.

Noom offers an alternative to standard dieting a tailored and distinctive approach to healthy living and weight loss. Through the integration of technology, psychology, coaching, and community support, Noom enables people to make long-lasting modifications to their lifestyle, habits, and health. Noom offers the resources, skills, and support you need to achieve your goals whether they be to improve nutrition, shed pounds, or form healthier habits.

An overview of Noom

Noom is a well-known wellness program that combines behavior modification strategies, individualized coaching, instructional materials, and community support to assist people in reaching their fitness and health objectives. Noom addresses the underlying behaviors, routines, and mentality that affect long-term success in order to adopt a holistic approach to weight loss and good living, in contrast to conventional diet plans that just emphasize calorie tracking or restrictive eating.

Essential Elements of Noom:

Behavioral Change: Noom's strategy is based on behavioral psychology and is centered on assisting users in creating durable lifestyle changes, better habits, and mental adjustments. The program's goal is to bring about long-lasting behavior change by highlighting the significance of tiny, regular behaviors.

Personalized Coaching: Noom gives customers access to a personal coach who will accompany them on their path and provide accountability, direction, and support. Coaches assist clients in overcoming obstacles, setting realistic objectives, and maintaining motivation. They are trained in behavior modification approaches.

Education and Awareness: To assist users in developing a deeper comprehension of psychology, fitness, and nutrition, Noom provides articles, interactive content, and educational resources. Users can make better decisions and build healthier habits by becoming more aware of the world and possessing more knowledge.

Food Tracking: Noom has a function called "Food Tracking" that uses color coding (green, yellow, and red) to classify foods according to their nutritional content and calorie density. This enables consumers to choose healthier foods without feeling constrained or undernourished.

Physical Activity: By establishing individualized activity objectives and offering advice on how to stay active, Noom helps users integrate physical activity into their everyday routines. It is believed that physical activity is crucial to general health and wellbeing.

Community Support: Noom provides a friendly environment for users to interact with one another, exchange stories, and acknowledge accomplishments. Support from the community can offer accountability, inspiration, and encouragement, making the path to improved health and fitness more pleasurable and long-lasting.

The Operation of Noom:

Assessment: First, users fill out a thorough questionnaire about their goals, lifestyle habits, preferences, and medical history. This data is utilized to generate a customized plan and personalize the program.

Goal Setting: Using the findings of the assessment, users collaborate with their personal coach to establish measurable objectives pertaining to behavior modification, physical activity, diet, and weight loss. The process of breaking down goals into small, doable steps boosts confidence and success.

Daily Assignments and Challenges: To assist users in reaching their objectives and encouraging behavior modification, Noom provides them daily assignments, challenges, and articles. These exercises concentrate on subjects like portion control, stress reduction, mindful eating, and creating healthy habits.

Tracking Progress: Using the Noom app, users may keep tabs on their weight, physical activity, food intake, and goal progress. To assist users in tracking their progress and staying on course, the app offers insights, visualizations, and comments.

Coaching and help: Individual users receive continuous help and direction from their personal coach, who follows up on a regular basis to offer encouragement, comments, and answers to queries. Coaches assist clients in navigating difficulties, overcoming roadblocks, and acknowledging accomplishments along the way.

Noom provides a thorough and individualized approach to healthy living and weight loss that takes into account the social, psychological, and behavioral aspects that affect outcomes. Through the integration of technology, psychology, coaching, and community support, Noom enables people to make long-lasting modifications to their lifestyle, habits, and health. Noom offers the resources, skills, and support you need to achieve your goals—whether they be to improve nutrition, shed pounds, or form healthier habits.

History and Evolution of the Noom Initiative

Two businessmen named Artem Petakov and Saeju Jeong launched the Noom program in

2008 with the goal of revolutionizing how people approach healthy living and weight loss. The idea behind Noom was their conviction that conventional diet plans frequently fell short in treating the psychological issues and underlying behaviors that lead to weight gain and make it difficult to maintain long-term improvements.

Using technology, cognitive behavioral therapy (CBT), and behavioral psychology, Petakov and Jeong set out to develop a holistic wellness platform that would enable people to make long-lasting lifestyle changes. They put together a group of specialists in technology, psychology, and nutrition to create a program that would include community support, educational materials, individualized coaching, and behavior modification strategies.

To make sure the Noom program was useful and effective, it was put through a rigorous testing, research, and improvement process. In order to incorporate evidence-based techniques for behavior modification and weight control into the program's structure, the founders worked with psychologists and researchers. Additionally, they made use of technology to develop a simple and easy-to-use app that would let users track their progress, access resources, and communicate with peers and their personal coach.

Noom's services have grown and changed throughout time to cover a broad range of health and wellness objectives, such as stress relief, fitness, nutrition, weight loss, and general well-being. Aiming to provide a comprehensive and individualized approach to health improvement, the program has attracted millions of users worldwide and gained significant reputation and appeal.

Noom is still innovating and improving its program today, taking into account user input, technological advancements, and new findings in the nutrition and psychology domains. Noom continues to lead the way in the digital health and wellness sector, enabling people to adopt long-lasting lifestyle changes and improving their quality of life.

CHAPTER TWO

Theoretical Framework and Methodology for Modifying Behavior

The Noom program's theory and method of behavior modification are based on the ideas of positive psychology, motivational interviewing, and cognitive behavioral therapy (CBT). Noom understands that changing one's behavior in a lasting way necessitates addressing the underlying attitudes, convictions, feelings, and routines that shape one's choices and actions.

Important Components of Noom's Behavior Change Methodology:

Noom places a strong emphasis on the value of self-awareness in comprehending one's own actions, routines, and driving forces. Users can better understand their eating habits, triggers, and obstacles to change by engaging in self-reflection.

Setting Goals: Noom assists users in establishing SMART (specific, measurable, achievable, relevant, and time-bound) objectives for physical activity, nutrition, weight reduction, and general well-being. Objectives are divided into more doable, smaller steps to boost motivation and achieve results.

Behavior tracking: With Noom's food journaling tool, users may monitor their daily caloric intake, amount of exercise, weight, and advancement toward their objectives. Users can become more conscious of their routines, trends, and advancements over time by recording their actions.

Education and Skill Development: Noom offers articles, interactive content, tests, and educational resources to assist users in gaining the knowledge, abilities, and decision-making techniques necessary to make healthy choices. Nutrition, mindful eating, stress management, portion control, and self-care are among the subjects covered.

Cognitive restructuring: Noom assists users in recognizing and disputing harmful attitudes, ideas, and behaviors around food, weight, and body image. Users can learn to reframe negative beliefs and cultivate a more positive and balanced mentality by using cognitive restructuring strategies.

Social Support: Noom creates a friendly environment where users may interact with one another, exchange stories, and get support and responsibility. Support from the community can offer inspiration, affirmation, and a feeling of inclusion during the process of changing one's behavior.

Personal Coaching: Noom gives its users access to a personal coach who may help with direction, accountability, and support. To assist clients in overcoming obstacles, maintaining motivation, and navigating difficulties, coaches employ research-backed strategies like goal-setting, motivational interviewing, and problem-solving.

Fundamentals of Successful Behavior Modification:

Noom places a strong emphasis on the value of taking tiny, regular steps and making little but steady progress toward objectives. Users gain self-assurance, momentum, and long-term success by concentrating on little adjustments.

Self-Efficacy: By offering encouraging comments, recognizing accomplishments, and emphasizing prior successes, Noom aims to increase users' self-efficacy, or confidence in their capacity to succeed. Increasing self-efficacy boosts drive and fortitude in the face of adversity.

Choice and Autonomy: Noom gives consumers the freedom to decide for themselves what is best for their health and wellbeing. Giving users autonomy, flexibility, and options makes them feel powerful and involved in the process of changing their behavior.

Sustainability: Noom encourages actions that will be long-lasting and sustainable. Noom promotes lifestyle modifications that enhance general health and well-being as opposed to emphasizing band-aid or rapid cures.

To assist people achieve long-lasting changes to their habits, lifestyle, and health, Noom places a high priority on self-awareness, goal-setting, education, social support, and individualized coaching. Noom gives individuals the tools they need to make significant and long-lasting changes in their life by addressing the behavioral, psychological, and emotional aspects of change.

Comprehending the Elements of the Noom Program

The Noom program's main elements are behavior modification, education, and support all of which are intended to help people reach their health and wellness objectives. Together, these elements offer a thorough and customized strategy for enhancing lifestyle and health. The Noom program consists of the following key components:

1. Tailored Guidance:

Assigned Coach: Every user is paired with a personal coach who supports, holds them accountable, and offers advice along the way.

Personalized Feedback: Coaches provide users with feedback that is tailored to their goals, obstacles, and level of progress.

Goal-setting: Coaches help clients define clear, attainable objectives and offer solutions for overcoming challenges.

2. Techniques for Changing Behavior:

Noom incorporates the concepts of cognitive behavioral therapy, or CBT, to assist users in recognizing and altering problematic ideas, attitudes, and actions linked to their health and well-being.

Motivational Interviewing: In order to promote a cooperative and empowering approach to behavior change, coaches employ motivational interviewing techniques to delve into the fundamental motivations, strengths, and values of their clients.

3. Food Recording and Monitoring:

Foods are divided into green, yellow, and red categories according to their nutritional value and calorie density, which helps consumers make better decisions.

Meal Logging: Participants record the amount of food they eat each day, keep tabs on their caloric intake, and track their advancement toward nutritional objectives.

Barcode Scanner: To rapidly log packaged goods and retrieve nutritional data, use the barcode scanner in the Noom app.

4. Resources for Education:

Articles & Quizzes: Through articles, quizzes, and interactive lessons, Noom offers instructional content on subjects including fitness, stress management, nutrition, and behavior modification.

Psychological Insights: In order to better understand and manage their health-related behaviors, users learn about the psychological aspects of behavior that influence them, such as habit formation, self-awareness, and motivation.

5. Community Assistance:

Group Support: Users become a part of an encouraging network of peers with comparable objectives, difficulties, and life experiences.

Group Challenges: Noom provides activities and challenges for groups of users to promote accountability, incentive, and companionship.

6. Monitoring Activities:

Physical Activity objectives: Users track their daily movement and exercise and create individualized objectives for their physical activity.

Integration with Fitness applications: To automatically log physical activity and sync data with the Noom platform, Noom connects with well-known fitness tracking applications and gadgets.

7. Tracking Progress:

Visualizations: To monitor progress in areas like weight loss, food intake, physical activity, and goal achievement, Noom offers charts and visualizations.

Feedback and Insights: Based on their progress data, users receive feedback and insights that assist them in recognizing trends, acknowledging accomplishments, and making necessary behavioral adjustments.

8. Availability:

Mobile App: Noom's mobile app lets users connect with their coach at any time and from any location, track their progress, and access resources.

Sync Between Devices: Information and progress are synchronized between PCs, tablets, and smartphones to provide a smooth user experience.

The Noom program empowers people to achieve long-lasting changes to their lifestyle and health by combining individualized coaching, behavior modification strategies, educational materials, peer support, and tracking tools. Through addressing the social, behavioral, and psychological components of behavior modification, Noom assists users in creating better habits, enhancing their wellbeing, and reaching their health objectives.

Noom's Method for Losing Weight

Noom approaches weight loss in a different and all-encompassing way that goes beyond conventional dieting techniques. The program helps people reach and maintain their weight loss goals by emphasizing psychology, education, support, and lasting behavior change. An outline of Noom's weight loss strategy is provided below:

1. Modification of Behavior:

Noom understands that in order to achieve long-term weight loss, it is necessary to address the underlying habits, mindsets, and behaviors that lead to overindulgence in food, inadequate nutrition, and sedentary lifestyles. The program helps participants create better habits and mindsets by utilizing evidence-based behavior change strategies like motivational interviewing, cognitive behavioral therapy (CBT), and positive psychology.

2. Tailored Guidance:

Every user is matched with a personal coach who helps them along the way with accountability, support, and direction in losing weight. Coaches help users overcome difficulties and barriers, provide personalized feedback, and help create goals. They enable individuals to achieve long-lasting changes by utilizing motivational interviewing techniques to investigate their values, abilities, and motivations.

3. Knowledge and Consciousness:

Noom offers articles, interactive material, educational resources, and tests to assist users learn more about nutrition, mindful eating, portion control, and behavior modification. As awareness and knowledge grow, users are better able to make decisions and build healthier behaviors.

4. Food Recording and Monitoring:

Using Noom's meal recording tool, users may keep track of their daily food intake, keep an eye on their calorie intake, and make better decisions. Users may make better balanced and nutrient-dense decisions by sorting foods into green, yellow, and red categories depending on their calorie density and nutritional worth.

5. a Community of Support:

Users can interact with others, exchange experiences, and get accountability and support in Noom's encouraging community. Users' motivation and sense of camaraderie are increased through group challenges, activities, and debates, which improves adherence and success.

6. Exercise:

Noom stresses the need of physical activity in addition to diet in reaching weight loss objectives. Users create individualized activity goals, monitor their movement and exercise, and get advice and inspiration to be active all day long.

7. Tracking Progress:

To assist users in tracking their progress and maintaining motivation, Noom offers charts, feedback, and visualizations. Users are able to track their food intake, exercise, weight loss, and goal success, which enables them to recognize their accomplishments and modify their behavior as necessary.

The core components of Noom's weight loss strategy include behavior modification, individualized coaching, information, encouragement, and progress tracking. Through tackling the psychological, behavioral, and social dimensions of weight reduction, Noom enables people to modify their lifestyles in a sustainable manner, accomplish their objectives, and enhance their general health and welfare.

Technology and the Noom App

Users can access all of the program's features, tools, and resources through the Noom app. It makes use of technology to give people looking to enhance their health and fitness a smooth, customized experience. An outline of the Noom app's main technological features is provided below:

1. Customized Dashboard:

Users see a personalized dashboard with their daily chores, goals, progress, and scheduled activities displayed as soon as they log in. The dashboard keeps the user organized and focused on their health objectives by giving them a quick overview of their trip.

2. Nutritional tracking and food journaling:

Users can log meals, track their daily food intake, and keep an eye on their nutritional intake with the app's food logging feature. Users may make better decisions by sorting foods into green, yellow, and red categories based on their nutritional worth and calorie density.

3. Barcode Reader:

By scanning the barcodes of packaged meals, users of Noom's barcode scanner may log them fast. With the help of this tool, users can easily measure their calorie consumption, precisely log items, and get nutritional information.

4. Monitoring Activities:

Users can use the app's activity tracking feature to monitor their movement, exercise, and physical activity. Individualized activity objectives can be defined, progress can be tracked, and advice on how to keep active all day long can be obtained.

5. Content for Education:

Users of Noom get access to a vast library of instructional materials, including articles, tests, and interactive content on subjects including psychology, behavior modification, fitness, and nutrition. The content of the app is tailored to the user's interests, progress, and goals.

6. Establishing and Tracking Goals:

Users can establish clear, attainable objectives for behavior modification, physical activity, diet, and weight loss. With the app, users may chart their accomplishments, keep an eye on their progress toward their goals, and modify their behavior as necessary.

7. Individual Coaching:

Through the app, customers may communicate with their personal coach and ask questions, get advice, and get help for whatever needs to be done along the way. To keep clients motivated and on course, coaches offer accountability, support, and feedback.

8. Community Assistance:

Users can interact with peers, take part in group activities, and share experiences through the Noom app. Users' sense of accountability, inspiration, and camaraderie are fostered by the app's community, which improves adherence and success.

9. Combining Fitness Equipment with Integration:

Noom's smooth integration with well-known fitness devices and applications enables users to sync their activity data. Users can track their exercise and physical activity on various platforms and devices thanks to this connectivity.

The Noom app uses technology to provide people who want to get healthier and feel better with a tailored, engaging, and encouraging experience. The app helps users reach their health goals and make durable lifestyle changes by combining features like activity monitoring, meal journaling, coaching, and community support.

Noom's Health Benefits

Noom prioritizes overall well-being over weight loss and provides its customers with a host of health benefits. The following are some of the main health advantages of the Noom program:

1. Long-Term Weight Loss:

Noom helps people reach and keep weight loss goals in a sustainable way by utilizing behavioral change methodologies, personalized coaching, and evidence-based strategies. Noom encourages long-lasting benefits by emphasizing long-term behavior modification as opposed to temporary solutions.

2. Better Eating

Noom provides customers with individualized assistance, educational materials, and food logging tools to help them adopt healthier eating practices and make better nutritional decisions. Users can enhance the quality of their diets overall by learning to choose nutrient-dense foods and balance their meals.

3. Enhanced Exercise:

By allowing users to create individualized activity goals, track their workouts, and offer encouragement and support, Noom helps users integrate physical activity into their daily routine. Engaging in regular physical activity enhances cardiovascular health, strength, and general well-being in addition to helping with weight management.

4. Modification of Behavior:

With its emphasis on cognitive restructuring, behavior modification strategies, and individualized coaching, Noom assists users in creating better routines and mentalities. Through addressing the underlying attitudes, thoughts, and behaviors that lead to weight gain, people can modify their lifestyle in a way that is sustainable.

5. Enhanced Sensitivity to Self:

Noom assists users in becoming more self-aware of their routines, triggers, and obstacles to change through self-reflection, goal-setting, and progress tracking.

CHAPTER THREE

Users who are more self-aware are able to take charge of their health and wellness and make more thoughtful decisions.

6. Enhanced Mental Well-Being:

To enhance users' mental health, Noom integrates stress reduction, mindfulness, and positive psychology into its platform. By mastering stress management methods, mindfulness exercises, and coping tactics, people can improve their mental toughness and general well-being.

7. a Community of Support:

With the help of Noom's community platform, users may interact with others in a safe space, exchange stories, and get accountability and support. Having a sense of community and belonging encourages motivation, involvement, and program adherence.

8. Reduced Risk of Long-Term Illnesses:

Noom assists users in lowering their chance of developing chronic illnesses like obesity, type 2 diabetes, heart disease, and some types of cancer by encouraging a balanced diet, regular exercise, and behavioral changes. Positive lifestyle adjustments can result in long-term gains in wellness and illness prevention.

Noom provides a holistic and individualized approach to health and wellness, emphasizing behavior modification, better nutrition, sustained weight loss, greater physical activity, elevated self-awareness, mental health, and social support. Noom gives users the tools they need to reach their objectives and lead happier, healthier lives by addressing various aspects of health.

Beginning to Use Noom

Noom's easy-to-follow setup process is intended to assist people in taking the first steps toward improved wellness and health. This is a detailed how-to for setting up Noom:

1. Register with Noom:

Go to the Noom website or get the Noom app from the Google Play Store or App Store.

Fill out the form when creating an account by entering your name, email address, and goals.

2. Finish the Evaluation:

You will be required to fill out an assessment after registering, which will collect data on your goals, lifestyle choices, past medical history, and preferences.

Noom uses the assessment to tailor the program to your unique requirements and preferences.

3. Create a Profile:

After finishing the assessment, create your profile by adding more details like your height, weight, gender, age, and level of activity.

Noom uses this data to determine your individual calorie and activity targets.

4. Make Contact with Your Own Coach:

Once your profile is created, you will be paired with a personal coach who will accompany you on your journey and offer accountability, support, and direction.

Spend some time getting to know your coach and talking about your preferences, goals, and any queries or worries you may have.

5. Examine the App:

Get acquainted with the features, resources, and tools of the Noom app.

Examine the instructional materials, tour the dashboard, experiment with the activity tracking and food logging tools, and visit the community platform.

6. Begin Recording Your Meals and Exercise:

Start recording your daily food intake and exercise using the activity tracking and food logging features of the app.

Try to keep a journal of everything you consume, including snacks and drinks, as well as any exercise or physical activity you perform during the day.

7. Establish Your Objectives:

Together with your personal coach, establish measurable objectives for behavior modification, physical activity, nutrition, and weight loss.

Divide your objectives into more achievable, smaller steps to boost motivation and success.

8. Participate in the Community:

Become a member of the Noom community to interact with other users, exchange experiences, and get support.

Engage in group discussions, activities, and challenges to improve accountability and motivation.

9. Remain Connected and Consistent:

Make a promise to yourself that you will continue to log, track, and set goals consistently.

To optimize your success, maintain contact with your personal coach, interact with the instructional materials, and take part in the Noom community.

It only takes a few minutes to get started with Noom: register, finish the assessment, get in touch with your coach, and browse the app's features. By being proactive in achieving your wellness and health objectives, you can position yourself to succeed with the Noom program.

Noom Guidance and Assistance

The program's essential elements are Noom coaching and support, which offers users individualized direction, accountability, and motivation all along their path to health and wellness. What to anticipate from Noom's coaching and assistance is as follows:

1. Tailored Guidance:

A committed personal coach is paired with each user to act as an accountability partner, mentor, and ally.

Coaches offer individualized advice, encouragement, and support based on the objectives, tastes, and difficulties of each client.

2. Individualized Conversation:

Through in-app messaging, users can communicate and receive support from their personal coach directly, facilitating continuous communication.

When a question, concern, or progress update comes up, coaches address it right away and offer advice and support as needed.

3. Setting Objectives and Monitoring Results:

Coaches assist clients in establishing clear, attainable objectives for behavior modification, physical activity, nutrition, and weight loss.

They keep tabs on users' advancement, acknowledge successes, and offer advice on how to get past roadblocks and stay on course.

4. Methods for Changing Behavior:

To assist clients in identifying and addressing change-related obstacles, coaches employ evidence-based behavioral change strategies like motivational interviewing and cognitive behavioral therapy (CBT).

They offer advice on how to overcome emotional eating, control cravings, form healthier habits, and make long-lasting lifestyle adjustments.

5. Resources and Education:

To help customers better comprehend diet, exercise, mindfulness, and behavior modification, coaches provide a wealth of educational tools, articles, tests, and interactive content.

By providing advice and insights based on users' achievements and obstacles, they enable people to take charge of their health and make educated decisions.

6. Accountability and Support:

In order to keep users motivated, involved, and consistent in their recording, tracking, and goal-setting endeavors, coaches offer accountability and assistance.

They foster a welcoming and nonjudgmental atmosphere where users can explore their journeys towards health and wellness by providing them with support, affirmation, and empathy.

7. Flexibility and Adaptability: Coaches modify their methods to fit the particular requirements, preferences, and situations of each client.

They guarantee that coaching sessions blend nicely with customers' daily routines and lifestyles by providing flexibility in scheduling and communication.

8. Constant Improvement: To keep current on the most recent findings, approaches, and best practices in behavior modification and health coaching, Zoom coaches participate in extensive training and ongoing professional development.

Their constant goals are to improve the application's usability, offer excellent customer service, and raise customers' satisfaction and success rates.

Users of Noom coaching and support receive individualized guidance, accountability, and motivation to help them achieve their wellness and health objectives. Through the implementation of evidence-based solutions, ongoing communication, and personalized support, Noom coaches enable individuals to make positive changes to their lifestyles that will last.

Monitoring Progress and Making Modifications

The Noom program's vital components of progress tracking and modification allow users to keep track of their progress, maintain accountability, and make the necessary adjustments to meet their wellness and health objectives. The Noom program's progress tracking and change process works as follows:

1. Tracking Tools: Noom gives users the ability to monitor their progress in a variety of categories, such as food, exercise, weight reduction, and behavior modification.

With the help of the app's tracking features, users can keep track of their daily food intake, calories consumed, physical activity, and progress made toward their goals.

2. Visualizations and Insights: To assist users in evaluating their progress and identifying patterns, trends, and areas for improvement, Noom provides charts, visualizations, and insights.

Users can track their food intake and exercise levels, analyze their weight loss progress over time, and get recommendations and feedback based on their data.

3. Goal Setting and Review: With the guidance of their personal coach, users set clear, attainable goals for food, exercise, behavior modification, and weight loss.

Coaches regularly evaluate their clients' progress toward their objectives, acknowledge their successes, and offer advice on how to overcome obstacles and stay on course.

4. Modifications & Adjustments: Coaches may suggest changes to users' objectives, behaviors, or strategies in response to their comments, challenges, and successes.

In collaboration with users, coaches pinpoint areas for improvement, adjust action plans, and set new objectives that align with their evolving needs and preferences.

5. Problem-Solving: Coaches assist users in problem-solving and developing strategies for getting beyond obstacles to their progress when they encounter difficulties or setbacks.

In order to help clients overcome obstacles, deal with setbacks, and maintain inspiration, coaches provide support, motivation, and useful solutions.

6. Flexibility and Adaptability: Nooom understands that consumers' needs and circumstances might change over time and that progress is not always linear.

In order to accommodate users' evolving preferences, schedules, and priorities, coaches provide flexibility and adaptation in changing goals, behaviors, and tactics.

7. Ongoing Assistance:

Throughout the Noom program, progress tracking and modifications are ongoing processes that guarantee participants receive ongoing support, direction, and encouragement.

In order to enhance their success and enjoyment with the program, coaches are available and responsive to the needs of their clients, providing customized assistance and adjustments as necessary.

The Noom program's core features, progress tracking and adjustments, let users keep track of their progress, pinpoint areas for growth, and make the necessary adjustments to reach their wellness and health objectives. Customers receive individualized support and coaching through ongoing tracking, evaluation, and adjustment processes to help them stay on course, get beyond challenges, and make long-lasting lifestyle improvements.

CONCLUSION

To sum up, Noom provides a comprehensive and customized approach to health and wellness that emphasizes support, food, exercise, sustainable behavior change, and physical activity. Users can access a wealth of resources, tools, and coaching to help them reach their goals and improve their general well-being through its innovative app-based platform.

Noom differs from other typical weight loss programs in that it places a strong focus on community support, education, individual coaching, and behavior modification techniques.

Through addressing the social, behavioral, and psychological aspects of health, Noom empowers people to improve their lives and adopt more sustainable lifestyles.

Noom provides the support, accountability, and motivation required for users to achieve their goals, whether they aim to enhance their general health, increase physical activity, improve nutrition, or lose weight. Noom's evidence-based methodology and dedication to user-centered treatment position it to have a long-lasting, substantial influence on people's health and wellbeing.

THE END